Achieving Flow

Paintball's Guide to Physical Fitness and Energy Boosting Nutrition

Table of Contents

Chapter 1. Introduction

Unleash your inner warrior and elevate your game with our Special Report: "Achieving Flow: Paintball's Guide to Physical Fitness and Energy Boosting Nutrition". Get ready to dive into an exciting exploration of skill enhancement and personal growth tailored specifically for the passionate paintball enthusiast. Not only will this report equip you with tools to boost your physical prowess, but it's also packed with insights on nutrition to rejuvenate your energy levels, all aimed at transforming you into an unequaled force on the battlefield. Paintball isn't just about strategy, it's a call to proficiency, endurance, and peak performance. Eager to get your heart racing and give your brainpower a jolt? Buy this Special Report today; it's your first step towards reaching the pinnacle of your paintball potential.

Chapter 2. Unlocking Your Paintball Potential: An Introduction

Paintball is so much more than a game. It's an exceptional fusion of physical athleticism, strategic precision, and mental agility. To unlock your full paintball potential, you must transform from the inside out. This transformation begins with a comprehensive understanding of the uniqueness of the sport. Paintball is a game where strategic flexibility and stamina are as crucial as a deadly aim.

2.1. Understanding the Game

Paintball is a sport that requires a unique blend of physical fitness, mental agility and tactical brilliance. Unlike other sports where the objective is clear and linear, paintball is dynamic with its objectives constantly shifting. One minute, you're pushing forward, the next, you're in retreat; one moment you're on defense, the next, you're on the offensive.

It's a sport of constant shifts and changes in tempo, requiring a player to adapt and adjust rapidly. Understanding these nuances goes a long way in enhancing your performance on the field. Knowledge fosters confidence, and confidence is a key driver in any sport.

2.2. Fitness for Paintball

Contrary to common perception, paintball is a physically demanding sport. Without appropriate physical conditioning, it's hard to keep up with the high-intensity stretches, sprints, diving and crawling often required in games.

You need to boost your cardiovascular endurance, muscular flexibility, agility, and strength. This can be achieved through a balanced regimen of aerobic exercises, strength training and flexibility-enhancing workouts. Exercises like running, skipping, plyometrics, bodyweight exercises, yoga and martial arts are beneficial.

2.3. Nutrition and Energy

Your diet plays a significant role in enhancing your performance on the field. A well-balanced diet not only fuels your body with essential nutrients, it also aids in quick recovery and sustained energy levels.

Understanding and implementing the right nutrition will help you maintain optimal energy levels, aid muscle recovery, enhance concentration and mental acuiteness, and boost overall physical performance. Make sure your diet is rich in carbohydrates for energy, lean proteins for muscle repair and recovery, and healthy fats for other vital bodily functions.

2.4. Mindset and Strategy

A winner's mindset and robust strategy are critical for success in paintball. Mental training techniques such as visualization, deep breathing and positive affirmation can significantly enhance your game performance. They help you handle pressure situations better, make more intelligent decisions, and stay calm when the game is not going your way.

It's equally important to understand the tactical aspect of the game. A well-thought-out strategy not only helps you respond effectively to different game situations, but it also gives your team a clear direction to follow.

2.5. Practicing Paintball Skills

As with any sport, practice is key to enhancing your paintball skills. This doesn't just mean repetitive shooting or sprinting. It means drilling all the key elements of the sport until they become second nature: shot accuracy, speed, stealth, tactics, communication and teamwork.

Professional players spend countless hours honing their skills and abilities. They understand that every small improvement makes a difference in the heat of the game. This understanding guides their approach to practice, ensuring that they never become complacent or take their skills for granted.

2.6. Essential Equipment and Gear

Good paintball performance is also dependent on having the right equipment. Your marker, hopper, air tank, paintball mask, and protective gear all play specific roles in your performance. Knowing precisely how to use, maintain and upgrade your gear can give you a distinct advantage on the field.

Overall, unlocking your full paintball potential requires a comprehensive approach that combines fitness training, nutrition, mental conditioning, tactical planning, practice, and equipment knowledge. It might seem daunting, but remember, every step forward, no matter how small, brings you closer to becoming an unequaled force on the battlefield.

So, gear up, step onto the paintball battlefield, and let every splatter of paint be a symbol of your unfaltering courage and indefatigable spirit. And above all, remember that the journey towards unlocking your paintball potential is not a sprint, but a marathon. It is not the destination, but the journey, that you should cherish. Let's get started!

Chapter 3. The Anatomy of a Paintball Warrior: Physical Conditioning

In a paintball match, victory isn't only decided by tactics and accuracy. A significant factor that predetermines your success on the battlefield is your physical condition.

3.1. Components of Physical Conditioning

Physical conditioning, at its core, incorporates strength, cardiovascular endurance, flexibility, balance, and speed. Let's dissect each component to understand its role and significance in the game of paintball.

1. Strength: Strength forms the foundation of your physical prowess. It adds power to your shots, throwing, crawling, and ducking movements. Targeting key muscle groups can help improve your overall performance. Particular attention should be given to the upper body since it plays a pivotal role in wielding a paintball gun and shooting accurately. Working out the lower body, mainly the thighs and the glutes, is also vital as running ducks, slides, and similar motions are invariably incorporated in each game.

2. Cardiovascular endurance: The length of a paintball match can be unpredictable. It relies on the size of the play area, the number of players, and the method of play. This uncertainty necessitates a high cardiovascular endurance level. Staying on the move is part and parcel of the paintball game. In a full-gear situation, a well-conditioned heart helps ensure optimal oxygen

supply to the muscles, reducing fatigue and enhancing performance.

3. Flexibility: Agile movements are crucial to evading shots and acquiring advantageous positions on the battlefield. Thus, conditioning exercises should include stretching routines to increase the range of body movements.

4. Balance: Paintball terrains can vary from woods to open fields to built obstacles, making balance an essential facet of fitness conditioning. It assists in steady aiming, rapid pivoting, and efficient maneuverability while lessening the risk of falls or stumbles.

5. Speed: The ability to quickly rush to covers, chase after enemies, or sprint away can be a game-changer. Speed plays a significant role in both offensive and defensive strategies making it a valuable trait to train.

3.2. Developing a Physical Conditioning Regime

Creating a physical conditioning regime relevant to paintball necessitates an understanding of the physical requirements of the match. Some of the exercises that can help build the necessary strength, agility, and endurance include:

1. Strength exercises: Include exercises like push-ups, pull-ups, and lateral raises to improve your upper body strength. Squats and lunges will enhance your lower body strength making you a formidable paintball player.

2. Cardio exercises: Running, cycling, or skipping can boost your cardiovascular endurance. Incorporating interval training, where periods of intense exercise are alternated with recovery periods, can replicate the stop-start nature of a paintball game.

3. Flexibility exercises: Incorporate stretches that target all the

major muscle groups. Yoga poses like the downward dog and triangle pose can also add to your flexibility.

4. Balance drills: Exercises like single-leg stance, standing knee hugs, and standing leg lifts can help improve your stability.

5. Speed drills: Plyometric exercises such as box jumps, burpees, and skater jumps, are excellent for building your speed.

3.3. Nutritional Support to Physical Conditioning

Proper nutrition is key to getting the maximum benefits from a physical conditioning program. Consuming a balanced diet rich in lean proteins, complex carbohydrates, and healthy fats is essential. Remaining well-hydrated is equally important, especially considering the long hours you may spend on the field.

Supplements can play a supportive role, but it is always advisable to have a professional guide you in understanding what your body needs.

In conclusion, strong physical conditioning is not just about improving your strength and endurance; it is about creating a harmonious and efficient linkage between all your body's components. It's about setting up a balance between your diet, training, and fitness goals. After all, an effective paintball warrior is a physical powerhouse, who, in addition to tactics and accuracy, leverages his physical supremacy to dominate the battlefield.

Chapter 4. Agility and Quick Reflexes: Essential Workout Routines

Rapid maneuvering, speed, and quick decision-making are the vital requisites of every paintball warrior. To excel in these areas, you must be commendably agile and possess extraordinary reflexes. Thus, the essential workout routines aimed at improving these facets are detailed ahead.

4.1. The Role of Agility in Paintball

Agility is the ability to move quickly and efficiently in any given moment. In the context of speedball, it's about how well and how quickly you can pivot, jump, dive, run, and maneuver within the space of a game. The more agile you are, the better you can dodge your opponents' marker shots, seize positions, and control the battlefield. Building agility involves working on strength, balance, and coordination. Let's dive into the different practices that can enhance these components.

4.2. Strength Training

Building maximum strength is the core of agility training, focusing mainly on your lower body and core. Your lower body provides the power for quick lateral movements, sprints, and jumps while your core keeps your body stable and balanced during these movements. Aim to perform these exercises three or more times a week for best results.

1. Deep Squats: Begin with a warm-up, then perform 3 sets of 15 reps of deep squats. It strengthens your thighs, buttocks, and

hips, leading to improved power in your leaps and dashes.

2. Bulgarian Split Squats: Execute 3 sets of 15 reps per leg which will help you with single-leg balance and strength.

3. Deadlifts: Perform 3 sets of 10 reps. This exercise adds strength to your lower body and core simultaneously, promoting stability during rapid movements.

4. Planks: Aim for three 1-minute planks to bolster your core's endurance.

4.3. Balance and Stability

Once you have strengthened your muscles, it's time to focus on enhancing your balance and stability. This skill is essential when you're negotiating uneven terrains or making challenging leaps.

1. Single-Leg Balance: Perform 3 sets of 1-minute holds per leg. This workout is a great way to improve your balance and stability.

2. Bosu Ball Squats: Practice Bosu ball squats for 3 sets of 15 reps. It forces your muscles to work harder to maintain balance, thereby improving your stability.

4.4. Coordination

Finally, the key to executing efficient movements is excellent coordination. This includes aligning your eyes and mind with your body's movements.

1. Ladder Drills: Consider investing in an agility ladder. It offers various drills that will boost your coordination and agility. Start with basic two-foot in-each-box exercises and then move up to more complex drills.

2. Ball Juggling: This exercise is not just fun but trains your brain and body to work together efficiently.

4.5. Boosting your Reflexes

Just as agility is crucial in paintball, so are quick reflexes. Rapid response times can mean the difference between victory and defeat as games often hinge on split-second decisions. Here are a few drills focused on this aspect.

4.6. Plyometrics

Plyometric exercises, also known as jump training or plyos, involve stretching a muscle and then contracting it quickly. These can promote quicker and more forceful contractions in the future, leading to improvements in speed and power.

1. Box Jumps: Begin with a lower height and gradually increase it as your ability improves. Execute 3 sets of 15.

2. Plyometric Push-Ups: Start in a classic push-up stance, lower your body then explode back up causing your hands to lift off the ground. Execute 3 sets of 15.

4.7. Reaction Training

This training is all about subjecting your body to unexpected situations and training yourself to respond quickly.

1. Ball Toss: Get a partner to randomly toss a ball towards you while you aim to catch it. Try increasing the speed and unpredictability as you progress.

2. Light Reaction Drills: There are several apps available that allow practicing light reaction drills. These work by providing visual stimuli that you must respond to as quickly as possible.

4.8. Flexibility

Lastly, maintaining a high level of flexibility assists in getting through tight spaces or jumping over obstacles without risk of injury. Incorporate stretching exercises into your workout routine.

1. Leg Stretches: Hold a forward lunge for about 30 seconds per leg. Follow it with hamstring stretch and seated groin stretch.

2. Upper Body Stretch: Practice chest stretch, shoulder stretch, and tricep stretch to ensure flexibility in your upper body.

3. Full Body: Execute yoga poses like downward dog, cobra pose, child's pose, standing forward bend for full body flexibility.

Consistency is key in training. Follow these exercises systematically and progressively and improve your agility and reflexes. Ultimately, the goal is not to turn you into a professional athlete but a formidable paintball player: agile, quick, and always ready for combat.

Chapter 5. Endurance is Key: Cardiovascular Training for Paintball

The exhilaration of sprinting across the field, the heart-pounding adrenaline from dodging your opponent's paints, the sheer satisfaction of claiming victory — these all point to a remarkably cardiovascular intense sport. Without a doubt, the game of paintball is as physically demanding as it is strategically gripping. This underscores the importance of robust endurance backed by a strong cardiovascular system.

The journey to optimizing your cardiovascular fitness for paintball begins with understanding the unique demands this sport imposes on your heart and lungs.

5.1. Unwinding the Cardiovascular Component in Paintball

Paintball isn't just about accuracy with the marker or spot-on strategy. The physical aspect of the game places significant stress on your cardiovascular system. It calls for short bursts of high-intensity activity such as running, dodging, crouching, and jumping, all of which invoke your heart and lungs to work harder.

Moreover, the adrenaline rush you experience during a game tends to accelerate your heart rate, amplifying the cardiovascular challenge the sport inherently poses. This prompts the need for targeted cardiovascular training to enable your body to handle and adapt to these conditions, consequently improving endurance, agility, speed, and recovery.

5.2. Designing Your Cardiovascular Training Regimen

Your cardiovascular training regimen should exhibit both versatility and specificity. Incorporate exercises that solicit similar movements and energy mechanisms utilized in paintball while employing various types of cardiovascular training to foster adaptability and overall cardiovascular health.

1. High-Intensity Interval Training (HIIT): This form of training demands bursts of high-intensity exercises followed by short periods of rest or lower-intensity activity. It parallels the burst-pause pattern characteristic of a typical game of paintball.

2. Continuous Cardiovascular Training: More prolonged, low-to-moderate intensity exercises like jogging, cycling, or swimming that condition your heart and lungs, improving their endurance.

5.3. Integrating High-Intensity Interval Training

HIIT workouts are beneficial for paintball because they mimic the sporadic nature of the sport's physical demands. Set up a HIIT routine as follows:

1. 5-minutes of warm-up: Light jogging or cycling

2. 30-seconds to 1-minute of high-intensity activity: Sprinting or burpees

3. 1-2 minutes of rest or light activity: Light walking or slow cycling

4. Repeat the high-intensity and rest combo 8-10 times

5. 5-minutes of cool-down: Stretching

5.4. Embedding Continuous Cardiovascular Training

Even though paintball is predominantly an anaerobic activity, incorporating steady-state aerobic exercises in your training ensures the efficiency of your cardiovascular system. You can pursue running, cycling, or swimming for around 30 to 60 minutes at a steady pace.

5.5. Monitoring Your Exercise Intensity

For optimal cardiovascular benefits, ensure to achieve the right exercise intensity. High-intensity intervals should push your heart rate to 80-90% of its maximum. During the rest periods or during steady-state cardio, aim to maintain the heart rate around 60-70% of its maximum. Use heart rate monitors or fitness watches to help with tracking.

5.6. Enhancing Recovery

Amid the hustle of enhancing your cardiovascular performance, recovery often gets sidelined. However, efficient recovery is vital to help your muscles and cardiovascular system recuperate and prepare for the next training session.

Ensure to:

1. Stretch before and after workouts

2. Hydrate efficiently

3. Take adequate rest

5.7. Complementing Cardio with Strength Training

Though cardiovascular exercises form an essential part of a paintball training program, it's equally important to integrate strength training. Paintball uses various muscle groups, and strengthening these muscles can lead to better performance and reduced injury risk. Complement cardio workouts with strength exercises targeting core, upper body, and lower body muscles.

By understanding the cardiovascular demands of paintball and rigorously adhering to a well-structured training program, you can significantly improve your in-game performance and resilience. Remember, a robust cardiovascular fitness not only fuels your triumphs on the battlefield but also empowers you with better health and fitness overall.

Chapter 6. Bodies in Motion: Flexibility and Injury Prevention

The human body is an exceptional machine, perfectly designed for motion. Its interconnected system of muscles, ligaments, and tendons allows for an astonishing range of movement. Irrespective of the sport, every athlete should maximize this range to enhance performance and prevent injury. In the world of paintball, flexibility plays a crucial role in agility and maneuverability. It facilitates fluid movements, decreases muscle tension, and imparts an edge in the game.

6.1. Understanding Flexibility

Flexibility is a measure of the range of movement in a joint or multiple joints that is affected by muscle length, joint integrity, and nervous system activity. It is essential to remember that flexibility is joint-specific, and its ranges can differ substantially among various joints.

The flexibility needed in a paintball game is directly related to functional movements involved in actions like crawling, ducking, diving, and shooting from various positions. Optimal flexibility helps lower the risk of injuries, decrease muscle imbalance and posture-related issues, and increases functional capabilities.

To measure your flexibility, physical tests like reach tests, bend-over tests, and rotational tests can be utilized. However, these should be performed under safety guidelines and professionals' supervision.

6.2. Incorporating Comprehensive Stretching Routines

Now that we know the significance of flexibility, let's dive into how to improve it. A comprehensive stretching routine, including static, dynamic, and functional stretches, can significantly enhance your flexibility.

1. **Static Stretching**: A stretching form that involves elongating a specific muscle or group of muscles to its fullest length and holding that position for about 15-60 seconds. E.g., the standing hamstring stretch.

2. **Dynamic Stretching**: Dynamic stretches involve functional based exercises that use sport-specific movements to prepare the body for performance. These are performed in a controlled, smooth, and deliberate manner to ensure muscle activation. Unlike static stretching, which elongates, dynamic stretching contracts and flexes muscles. E.g., the arm and leg swings.

3. **Functional Stretching**: This stretch style incorporates functional movements, focusing on the agility and balance needed on the field. Eg., the walking lunges with a twist.

Regularly engaging in these stretching exercises will boost your overall flexibility and perceptibly improve your paintball game.

6.3. The Importance of a Warm-up Routine

Before any stretching routine, it is crucial to begin with a warm-up. A good warm-up routine activates your cardiovascular system, raising your body temperature and increasing blood flow to your muscles. This routine decreases your risk of injuries and improves your performance level.

Some recommended warm-up exercises include a brisk walk, light jogging, jumping jacks, or body-weight exercises. Generally, the warm-up should be a lighter version of the activity you are about to perform and must be carried out for about 5-10 minutes.

6.4. Injury Prevention

Paintball's high intensity, coupled with an unpredictable terrain, can lead to injuries ranging from minor sprains to more severe problems like ACL tears or spinal injuries. Therefore, it's imperative to prioritize injury prevention in your training routine.

Aside from flexibility exercises and warm-ups, other injury prevention strategies include strength training, incorporating balance exercises into your routine, and ensuring proper hydration and nutrition.

1. **Strength Training**: Improve muscle health and resilience by focusing on the significant muscle groups you use in paintball, including the core, legs, and arms. Activities like resistance training, weight lifting, or plyometrics can be beneficial.

2. **Balance Exercises**: Performing balance-focused exercises, such as single leg stands or yoga, can improve your stability, decrease your risk of falls, and improve muscular balance and joint stability.

3. **Hydration & Nutrition**: Hydrating properly and eating a balanced diet fuels your muscles and aids recovery. Drink adequate fluids before, during, and after the game. Consuming foods rich in protein and complex carbohydrates aids in muscle repair and energy replenishment.

In conclusion, flexibility and injury prevention hold profound importance for a paintball warrior. Flexibility enhances your performance, while attention to injury prevention ensures longevity in the sport. Regular stretching, strength training, balance exercises, and excellent nutrition will fortify your body, preparing it for the intense excitement that paintball entails. As you level up your flexibility, you will notice a notable edge in your agility and speed, taking you a step closer to the pinnacle of your paintball prowess.

Chapter 7. Fueling the Warrior: Foundations of Energy-Boosting Nutrition

In order to truly boost and maintain your energy levels for the physical exertion required in paintball wars, a solid understanding and application of beneficial nutrition is critical. In this section, we will be exploring the cornerstones of energy-based nutrition; ranging from the basic macros and micros to understanding meal timings and hydration.

7.1. The Macro-Universe

Macronutrients, otherwise known as 'macros', comprise your primary food groups: carbohydrates, proteins, and fats. In terms of energy-boosting nutrition, these are the fuel your body will use to empower your paintball performance.

Carbohydrates are your body's preferred energy source. While carbs often suffer from an ill repute in the weight loss world, for athletes and paintball players alike, it's a significant and beneficial aspect. They break down into glucose, fueling muscles and brain processes. Whole grains, fruits, and vegetables are excellent sources of complex carbohydrates that provide sustained energy release.

Proteins have a vital role in muscle repair and building, which indirectly contribute to energy via improved endurance. Include lean meats, dairy, eggs, and plant-based options like legumes, nuts, and seeds in your diet.

Fats, particularly unsaturated ones, can provide long-term energy reserves, essential in endurance sports. Healthy fat sources include olive oil, avocados, nuts, seeds, and fatty fish.

7.2. The Mighty Micros

While macronutrients form the basis of our diet, micronutrients also play a crucial role. They are essential for overall wellbeing, including energy production and muscle performance.

B-Vitamins are integral in converting nutrients into energy. Rich sources include whole grains, meats, dark leafy vegetables, and fruits.

Iron directly influences energy by contributing to the proper function and formation of red blood cells, which carry oxygen to muscles. Find it in protein-rich foods like lean meats and dark green vegetables.

Potassium and Magnesium contribute to nerve signaling and muscle contractions, translatable to shooting stability in a paintball match. They are abundant in fruits, vegetables, and dairy products.

7.3. Timing is Everything

An adequately timed eating schedule is integral in maintaining consistent energy levels. Aim to eat balanced meals every 3-4 hours with an emphasis on complex carbs, adequate protein, and healthy fats.

Pre-game, it's ideal to consume a meal about 2-3 hours before the start, focusing on carbohydrates for readily available energy. During a paintball match, it might be challenging to consume something substantial. However, energy-rich snacks such as bananas or nuts can form an excellent pick-me-up.

Post-game, refill your tanks with a mix of proteins for muscle recovery, carbohydrates to replenish glycogen stores, and water to rehydrate.

7.4. Hydration for the Game

Proper hydration cannot be overstated for optimal performance. Dehydration hampers both physical prowess and mental acuity essential on the paintball battlefield. Alongside plain water, also consider drinks with electrolytes to replace minerals lost in sweat during the game.

7.5. Tailoring Your Diet

Every player is unique, and what works for one may not work for another. It's important to note distinct factors such as age, gender, metabolic rate, health, and intensity of play in designing a suitable nutrition plan. Same goes for potential food allergies or intolerances.

In conclusion, fueling your inner paintball warrior is a delicate balance of understanding and implementing the principles of macronutrients, appreciating the power of micronutrients, using meal timing to your advantage, and maintaining optimal hydration levels. With knowledge and discipline, you can effectively boost your performance to reach unparalleled heights on the battlefield.

Chapter 8. Game On: Pre-Game Nutritional Strategies

To achieve peak performance in paintball, it's crucial to fuel your body appropriately before every game. The right diet not only enhances stamina and endurance but also improves focus and reaction time. Our bodies function best with a balanced energy source that includes carbohydrates, proteins, and fats, accompanied by adequate hydration.

8.1. Carbohydrate Loading

Carbohydrate loading, popular amongst endurance athletes, proves effective in increasing your energy levels during a strenuous paintball battle. Consuming complex carbohydrates, like whole grains, fruits, and vegetables, 1-3 days prior to the game replenishes glycogen reserves in your muscles, providing you sustained energy when you need it.

Food Source	Amount	Carbs
Whole Grain Bread	1 slice	15 gms
Brown Rice	1 cup	45 gms
Sweet Potato	1 medium	30 gms
Bananas	1 medium	30 gms
Blueberries	1 cup	20 gms

Remember, pairing complex carbohydrates with proteins can aid muscle repair and recovery while decreasing muscle fatigue.

8.2. Pre-Game Meal

Plan your pre-game meal 2-3 hours before the game. It should primarily consist of low-glycemic complex carbohydrates for sustained energy and moderate protein for muscle recovery. Avoid fatty foods as they're harder to digest and could disrupt the game.

Food	Carbs	Protein	Fat
Chicken Breast Sandwich (Whole Wheat Bread)	60g	35g	10g
2 Hard Boiled Eggs with 1 medium Sweet Potato	30g	13g	10g
Greek Yogurt with Granola and Berries	45g	20g	5g

Don't forget to hydrate! Sip water along with your meal to promote better digestion and prevent dehydration later.

8.3. Game-Day Hydration

Regardless of the weather, hydration is key. Dehydration could result in impaired cognitive functioning, slower reaction times, and reduced endurance. Start hydrating from the moment you wake up, aiming for at least 500ml-1000ml before the game.

Hydration Level	Water Intake
Low Intensity Game	1.5 - 2 Liters

Hydration Level	Water Intake
High Intensity Game	2 - 3 Liters
Hot Weather Game	3 - 4 Liters

Remember to drink at regular intervals during the game to maintain optimal hydration levels, especially when playing under the sun.

8.4. Quick Energy Boosts

Sometimes, the paintball game stretches beyond expected timeframes, and you need a quick pick-me-up. In such cases, opt for a quick-digesting carbohydrate source like a banana, oranges, or energy gels. This gives your body immediate fuel to maintain concentration and energy levels.

Food	Amount	Quick Energy
Banana	1 medium	Yes
Orange	1 small	Yes
Energy Gel	1 Pack	Yes

Though these strategies will help you get fully equipped nutritionally for an epic paintball battle, remember everyone's body is unique. Listen to your body, test different combinations, and see what makes you feel the best and perform optimally. After all, nothing should come between you and your game!

Chapter 9. In the Trenches: Hydration and Nutrition During Play

When it comes to peak performance in paintball, focusing solely on shooting precision and navigational prowess is a common pitfall. While it's undeniable that these skills are integral, it's equally important to remember your nutrition and hydration status during play. You're squaring off against both your opponents and physical exhaustion on the battlefield, and these two components, hydration and nutrition, significantly minimize fatigue and enhance endurance, helping you get the upper hand.

9.1. Hydration Tactics

Hydration is the first line of defense against energy drain in the field, especially because heavy bouts of physical activity like paintball can make you lose an incredible amount of water through sweat. Dehydration alters your bodily functions, affects your cognitive capabilities, and slows your reaction time. Certainly, none of these are conducive to claiming victory on the paintball field.

9.2. Keeping Up with Water Intake

Aim to drink about 500 milliliters of water 2-3 hours before a game. This helps to prime your body for the vast amounts of water loss it's about to experience. Then, during the play itself, try to sip water at regular intervals, preferable at every break between games. Drinking around 150-200ml of water every 20-30 minutes of intense play will help you maintain optimally hydrated status.

But how do you remember to hydrate amidst the thrill of the game?

Implementing water breaks strategically throughout the play schedule is a great way to ensure players maintain this crucial hydration level. The breaks not only serve as reminders to hydrate, but also provide much-needed respite during sessions of high-intensity gameplay.

9.3. Hydration Indicators

Determining when you're hydrated or approaching a state of dehydration can be boiled down to two primary indicators - urine color and thirst level.

Your urine's version of an "amber traffic light", excessively yellow or gold urine, is a warning sign that you're either dehydrated or close to it. A better state of hydration would result in light yellow to clear colored urine.

"Thirst" isn't a particularly accurate indicator as your body only signals thirst when it's already somewhat dehydrated. However, if you're not accustomed to drinking copious amounts of water, it may be the motivation you need to gulp down those much-needed glasses of H2O.

9.4. Recognizing Dehydration

Fatigue, dizziness, muscle cramps, and headaches are common symptoms of dehydration. In extreme cases, you may even feel nauseous or faint. If you find yourself experiencing any of these signs, it's crucial to take a break, drink some water and maybe a little bit of sports drink to replenish the electrolytes.

9.5. Fluids Beyond Water

When you sweat, your body loses more than just water - it loses essential electrolytes like sodium, potassium, and magnesium. These mineral salts play vital roles in fluid balance, nerve function, and muscle contraction.

In exceptionally heated or lengthy games, you might benefit from incorporating sports drinks and coconut water, both packed with these essential electrolytes. These can be a secondary source of hydration to regular water intake, albeit focused on replenishing lost electrolytes.

9.6. Nutrition Playbook

While staying hydrated is non-negotiable, nourishing your body with the right nutrients is the other half of a perfect defense against exhaustion. Feeding your body with the right fuel will optimize your energy stores, ensuring you can sprint, dodge, aim, and shoot with accuracy and speed throughout the game.

9.7. Pre-Game Fueling

Carbohydrates are the body's primary source of energy. The night before a big game, consider loading up on nutrient-dense carbohydrate-rich meals to help optimize glycogen stores in your muscles, ensuring your energy tank is filled to the brim.

Examples of such meals could be whole grain pasta with lean protein like grilled chicken, and a side of vegetables. Whole grains release glucose into your bloodstream gradually, ensuring a steady stream of energy.

9.8. Keeping Energy Levels Up During Play

During the play, refueling is essential. Consuming a mix of high-fiber carbohydrates and lean proteins can provide slow-release energy that can maintain your vigor throughout the day. Nuts, bananas, or even a granola bar are good choices for a nourishing snack amidst the intense gameplay. Remember, smaller more frequent meals prevent overwhelming your digestive system during strenuous activity.

9.9. Maintaining Protein Intake

While carbohydrates ensure constant energy availability, protein assists in muscle recovery, preventing damage during strenuous physical activities. Beef jerky, protein bars, or a handful of almonds can be quick, hassle-free protein boosts during the game.

9.10. A Note on Timing

It's crucial to time your intake correctly to maximize nutritional benefits while avoiding digestive turmoil. Aim to consume these energy-boosting snacks roughly 20-30 minutes into each break to allow your body ample time for digestion before resuming play.

In the end, nutrition and hydration during play boil down to two essential ideas: continual water intake and strategic fueling with nutrient-rich snacks. Keep these in mind, and you'll maintain the energy and sharpness needed to dominate the paintball battlefield.

Chapter 10. A Warrior's Recuperation: Post-Game Refueling and Recovery

Physical exertion is an inherent part of any sport, and paintball is no exception. As a player, you're constantly on the go: sprinting, dodging, ducking, and diving — all while strategizing and aiming under high-stress conditions. Not unlike a warrior in combat, your body and mind are pushed to their limits. This calls for a specific focus on recuperation and post-game refueling, which will help restore your energy, aid muscle recovery, and prepare you for the next battle.

10.1. Refueling 101: Understanding Energy Replenishment

Working out the intricate logistics of a game drains you, both physically and mentally. Hence, there's a need to refuel. Firstly, understand that the body derives energy from three primary nutrients: carbohydrates, proteins, and fats. Their ratio in your diet can be fine-tuned to maintain, lose, or gain weight, with the understanding that picking the right types of each is crucial.

Carbohydrates should be primarily complex carbs (like whole grains, fruits, and vegetables), providing a steady energy release. Proteins, preferably lean (like chicken, fish, lentils, or tofu), aid in muscle repair, while healthy fats (like avocados, nuts, or olive oil) provide a dense energy source and are crucial for vitamin absorption and hormone production.

10.2. Assessing Your Needs: Macro & Micronutrients

Your nutrient requirements largely depend on the intensity and duration of your game. However, a ballpark figure for a 150-pound paintball player who plays a full day might burn around 1500 to 2000 calories. Aim to fill these back in with a ratio of 50% carbohydrates, 30% protein, and 20% fats.

Now, speaking of micronutrients, paintball warriors must focus on vitamins, minerals, and water above ingested food. These play a pivotal role in maintaining your body's operational efficiency. Hydration is fundamental. Couple your post-game meal with enough water to replenish your body's lost fluids.

10.3. Eating Timing: When and What to Eat?

Upon the game's conclusion, aim to eat within the first 30 minutes to an hour. This window is when your body's ability to refill its glycogen store is at its highest. A mix of lean protein and simple, fast-digesting carbs is pivotal here. A protein shake with a banana could offer an easy and quick solution.

An hour or two post-game, a more substantial meal should be consumed. Ideally, this might include a lean protein source, a variety of vegetables for additional nutrients and fiber, some complex carbs, and a small portion of healthy fats.

10.4. Post-Game Hydration: More Than Just Water

Not only water but electrolytes lost through sweat need to be replenished. Just remember that not all sports drinks are created equal. Look for options low in processed sugars. A good choice could be drinks that include a balance of electrolytes, including sodium and potassium.

10.5. Importance of Sleep: Your Natural Recovery Tool

Sleep is integral to recovery. During this time, your body experiences several restorative processes such as muscle repair and memory consolidation. Aim for 7 to 9 hours of quality sleep per night to maximize these benefits. You can deepen your sleep by reducing pre-bed screen time, keeping a cool and dark room, and maintaining a consistent sleep schedule.

10.6. Recovery Workouts: Low-Intensity, High Return

Active recovery routines, like yoga or walking, could be of immense benefit after a game. They assist in enhancing blood circulation, which in turn accelerates the healing of your muscle sore. Remember, the goal here isn't to exhaust but to rejuvenate.

10.7. Listen to Your Body: Know When to Rest

Finally, it's key to listen to your body's signals. Overtraining or burnout are common among athletes, and can drastically reduce performance, even lead to injuries. Ensure you balance your play time with adequate downtime, allowing your body the chance to fully recover.

Recuperation is an art, as much as it is a science. Never overlook its importance in your paintball journey. The right balance of nutrition, hydration, rest, and recovery techniques will restore your energy, speed up muscle repair, and set you up for the challenges of your next game. Prepare yourself to be not just a warrior, but a discerning one, ready to fight another day with renewed vigor and resilience. Remember - you are what you eat, drink, and how well you recharge.

Chapter 11. Mastering the Flow: A Comprehensive Fitness and Nutrition Checklist for Paintball

Getting in the zone, experiencing 'flow,' that intrinsic state where concentration is at its peak, and every action seamlessly ties into the next is vital for mastery in any sport, and paintball is no exception. This chapter aims to unravel step-by-step strategies, exercises, and dietary guidelines that not only enhance your paintball performance but also elevate your overall fitness and energy levels.

11.1. Boosting Fitness: The Flexible Paintball Exercise Plan

Impeccable fitness in paintball doesn't solely revolve around one exercise; it's about covering all the bases - agility, speed, endurance, strength, and flexibility.

A comprehensive fitness plan for a paintball enthusiast should include:

1. Cardio: Running, jogging, swimming, cycling, and HIIT are great for developing a robust cardiovascular foundation. These exercises boost lung capacity, improve heart health, and increase overall stamina, vital to sustain the energy required in a demanding match of paintball. A 30-minute high-intensity interval training (HIIT) three to four times a week can do wonders for your endurance levels.

2. Strength Training: Incorporate exercises targeted at the back, legs, and core muscles. Squats, lunges, push-ups, pull-ups, and

deadlifts not only fortify muscle strength but also enhance your ability to carry heavy equipment, sprint, crouch, and maintain stability during the game. Embrace a routine with these exercises at least twice a week.

3. Flexibility: Stretching both pre and post workout helps prevent injuries, improve coordination, and boost performance greatly. Focus on dynamic stretching before the game and static stretching afterwards to promote muscle recovery.

4. Speed and Agility: Incorporate agility ladders, side to side jumps, burpees, tuck jumps, shuttle runs in your routine. These enhance defensive maneuverability, and sprinting abilities needed for quick retreats or surprise attacks.

Remember, regularity is key. Consistency in your efforts becomes evident in your performance during the paintball match.

11.2. Pivotal Performance Nutrition: What to Eat for Enhanced Energy

Food is the fuel that runs the machine we call our body. But, what should this fuel constitute to ensure top-tier performance on the field?

1. Carbohydrates: As our body's main energy source, carbohydrates should be consumed in abundance before and following a match or workout. Whole grains, fruits, vegetables, and legumes are excellent sources of complex carbohydrates which provide a steady energy supply.

2. Protein: Vital for muscle repair and growth, proteins should be taken post-workout or match. Lean meats, dairy, eggs, and plant-based proteins like legumes and tofu are excellent choices.

3. Healthy Fats: Fats are an essential energy source, especially in endurance activities like paintball. Avocados, nuts and seeds,

fatty fish, and olive oil contribute good fats to your diet.

4. Hydration: Staples in any sport, water and sports drinks replenish fluids lost through sweat during a strenuous match. Aim for consistent hydration before, during, and after the game.

To keep you on track, prepare a weekly meal plan considering your calorie and nutrient needs, based on your body type, weight, and activity levels.

11.3. Fortifying Through Supplements

In addition to a balanced diet, supplementation can benefit your performance by fulfilling any potential nutrient gaps. Always consult a healthcare provider before beginning any supplement regimen.

1. Multivitamins: These provide a broad range of essential vitamins and minerals, supporting overall health and wellbeing.

2. Omega-3s: These healthy fats aid in cardiovascular health and reduce inflammation, assisting in recovery post matches.

3. Protein Powders: An easy way to meet your increased protein needs. They support muscle growth and recovery.

4. BCAA: Branched-chain amino acids help in muscle recovery and reduce muscle soreness post-workouts.

11.4. Mental Fitness: Building the Mind-Muscle Connection

Physical fitness is not all there is to mastering flow. Mental strength, focus, and the mind-muscle connection are integral components of this state of perfect synchrony.

1. Meditation and Visualization: Meditate daily to reduce stress, improve focus, and clarity of thought. Adding visualization to your meditation, imaging game scenarios and formulating strategies can significantly improve your performance.

2. Mindfulness: Incorporate mindfulness in your training, focusing wholly on the task at hand. This aids in bettering the mind-body connection, crucial in sports performance.

3. Sleep: An often overlooked, but crucial aspect of fitness and performance; ensuring quality sleep is a must for both physical recovery and mental sharpness.

Understanding and consistently improving your physical fitness, mastering your nutritional needs, and strengthening the mental aspect will indisputably put you in a favorable position to achieve flow on the paintball battlefield. Utilize this knowledge to your advantage and relentlessly elevate your game.